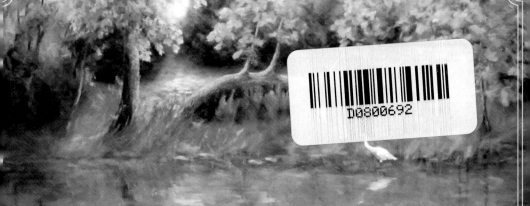

BRINGING
Kindness
TO
MEDICINE

STORIES *from the* PRAIRIE

JEROME W. FREEMAN, MD

Other Books by Jerome W. Freeman, MD

The Call to Care
(Co-editor and author with Arthur Olsen,
Mary Auterman and Ron Robinson)
The Colors of Care (essays)
Come and See (essays)
Easing the Edges (poetry)
Something at Last (poetry)
Starting from Here (poetry)

BRINGING
Kindness
TO
MEDICINE

STORIES *from the* PRAIRIE

JEROME W. FREEMAN, MD
SHEILA AGEE, MFA

Heroic Yes! Productions LLC, Publisher
San Diego, California

Bringing Kindness to Medicine:
Stories from the Prairie
All Rights Reserved.
Copyright © 2014 Jerome W. Freeman, MD
v2.0

ISBN: 978-0-578-12577-0

Published by
Heroic Yes! Productions LLC
www.HeroicYesProductions.com

Library of Congress Control Number: 2013911811

PRINTED IN THE UNITED STATES OF AMERICA

This book is dedicated to
the teachers and patients who have
helped fashion my life in medicine

More Praise for *Bringing Kindness to Medicine* by Dr. Freeman

"In healthcare today, there is considerable focus on issues such as access, safety, efficiency and quality. Rarely do you hear mention in the context of priorities and professionalism, the simple notion of kindness. Yet, it is fundamental to caring and when absent in a clinical encounter, even with a "good" outcome, the patient may feel diminished. *Bringing Kindness to Medicine* brings to life stories that remind us of the human condition of vulnerability and fragility and the abundant opportunity we have as caregivers to extend kindness not only to our patients and their families but also to our colleagues and to ourselves. Being kind doesn't take more time. It does require being intentional and unwavering in our commitment. Dr. Freeman suggests that perhaps clinicians need to be challenged to view their profession as a solemn calling. Indeed this would make medicine worthy of being called a noble profession. I would love to see this book get in the hands of students in the health professions as well as practicing clinicians."

Mary Jo Kreitzer, PhD, RN, FAAN
Founder and Director, Center for Spirituality & Healing
University of Minnesota

Praise for *The Colors of Care: What are Those Doctors Thinking* by Dr. Freeman

"This collection is a delight to read. Dr. Freeman has mastered the art of the short personal essay in which he writes about a single observation or incident that sheds light on an aspect of the human condition. In these essays Dr. Freeman employs his medical sensibility to imbue new meaning to a '58 Ford pickup, his father-in-law's garden, Andrew Wyeth's paintings, and an idiosyncratic bolo tie. He also reflects on patients and the foibles of medical practitioners. In every case his gentle wit and clear writing welcome the reader. And if the reader is anything like me, he or she immediately wants to join this master storyteller, as if they were sitting together on the front porch, and listen. I don't know whether the layperson will learn what 'those doctors' are thinking, but he or she will certainly learn—and be charmed and enlightened by—what this doctor is thinking."

Jack Coulehan, MD
Author of *Medicine Stone*
Editor of *Chekhov's Doctors*

"This might be the most edifying book you'll read this year. Through short reflections on his experience, Dr. Freeman brings one face to face with the human aspects of medicine. I highly recommend this collection to physicians, patients, and anyone who will ever be either."

Mark G. Kuczewski, PhD
Director, Neiswanger Institue for Bioethics & Health Policy
Stritch School of Medicine, Loyola University Chicago

Contents

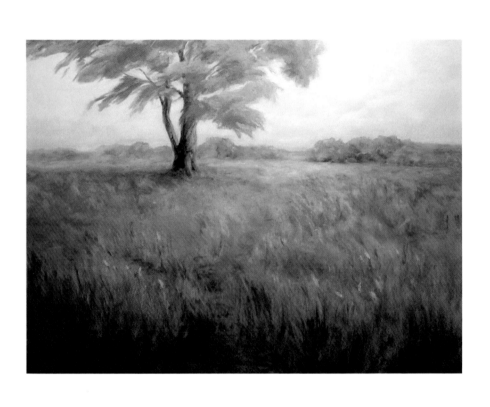

Foreword

From the time we were children, we've known about kindness. We respond to kindness and treasure it. We talk about it. Often the stories we tell one another revolve around kindness or the lack of it. Kind action can influence our behavior and have a ripple effect beyond our imaginations.

Because I have been a practicing physician for over thirty years, I most commonly think of kindness in a medical context. My world view is stitched together with narratives of illness.

Each of us knows when we have been treated kindly or unkindly. There is much tenderness and goodwill in the lives around us. And, of course, there can be treachery as well. Mostly, we learn kindness through the examples we encounter and the stories we share.

The person each of us becomes develops slowly. A compelling memoir could take the shape of a kindness chronicle. How intriguing to learn of the collective kindnesses that fashion an individual's life in medicine. We learn from our mentors, colleagues, students and patients. We learn from the actions we take, good and bad. Such a kindness chronicle could highlight the compounding effect and enduring legacy of individual acts of kindness, revealing a widening ripple over a community and beyond.

The narratives in this book are not a comprehensive chronology. Rather, they should be viewed as an amble, a leisurely stroll through nearby fields of kindness. Sheila Agee's artwork of the prairie complements the text. Pictures from a metropolitan area, perhaps an economically depressed inner city, could have worked as well. Images of kindness can be seen or imagined anywhere. She has chosen scenes that have the unifying element of a path or trail. The metaphor of a path has allure and promise. It can imply both choice and mystery. A path dipping out of view may hint at remorse. Sometimes the opportunities we have to extend a kindness are fleeting. Over the years, I've found that we aren't always given the chance to retrace our steps and return the way we came.

One: Opportunity

There is not enough kindness in medicine. I know. It's the world I live in most days. There is plenty of science and technology. Sophisticated tests and mind-boggling therapies abound. Sometimes desperately ill people are pulled back from the brink and given, as it were, a second life.

But all too often, the marvelous powers of medicine are not accompanied by the soft touch of kindness. Some clinicians, at times, seem to pride themselves on both the superiority of their technical abilities and their calm detachment from those being treated. It can be tempting to dabble in the fray of illness care while remaining remote from its consequences.

To clarify, my use of the term "medicine" refers to everyone engaged in illness care. Some may favor the terms "clinician" or "provider" as being more generic or inclusive. Many disciplines interact with patients, especially in the hospital setting. Physicians, nurses, social workers, phlebotomists, pharmacists and radiology technicians can all have a personal impact on the care a patient receives.

Basic kindness seems to be insufficiently emphasized by each of these groups and others in healthcare. Often encouraging words or a gentle touch are lacking. Certainly there are abundant excuses and justifications for essentially unkind behaviors. Those who provide illness care may feel too busy, too stressed, too preoccupied or too important. Remarkably, our society has, for the most part, come to expect and accept such rationalizations. A patient may struggle to even articulate what is hoped for. Perhaps a patient's uncertain expectations work to magnify the impact of every kindness that is experienced.

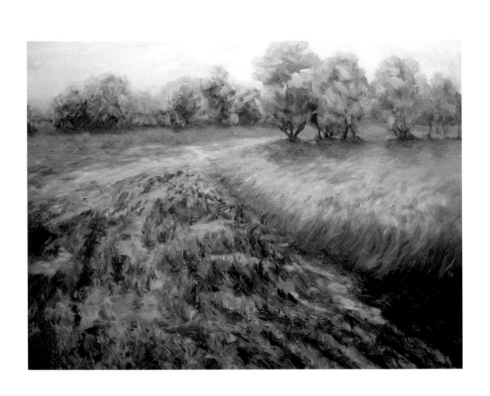

Two: Tribute

A nursing (and physician) story comes to mind. My office nurse and I had several patients to see in the hospital before beginning clinic. The day seemed to portend many obligations and insufficient time.

We arrived at a patient's room in a time of crisis. He had just rushed to the bathroom with diarrhea and sat down on the toilet without lifting the lid. Having been hastily bathed by the hospital aides, he was now sitting on the edge of his bed and adamantly refusing to go to the radiology department. The office nurse had known this patient for some time. She quickly moved around me and the two aides who were warily considering his new intransigence. Putting her hand on his arm, she patiently explained to him why it was important for him to have his x-ray done. He nodded reluctantly and asked her if she'd help him put his underpants on. "You won't be embarrassed, will you?," he asked shyly. She deftly slipped his shorts over his swollen legs and then stood close enough for him to lean against her as she pulled the shorts all the way up.

The patient then sat firmly down again on the bed. "I need to wash my hands first," he declared. Acting as if she had all morning (while I furtively glanced at my watch and thought of patients waiting at the clinic), the office nurse filled a shallow basin with warm water. She sat beside him and gently washed his hands, while he gazed at her solemnly. He seemed to bask in her attention as she carefully dried his hands before expertly assisting his wobbly effort to stand and pivot into the wheelchair. The aides and I were so mesmerized by the force and dignity of this interaction that none of us even moved forward to assist with the transfer.

On that day, she was just being a nurse, I suppose. Seemingly without forethought, she intervened to do what was needed to comfort this person. For many patients, there are times when high tech medicine is simply not enough. On such occasions, the patient is not asking for more than we can give, but for what we may not think to offer.

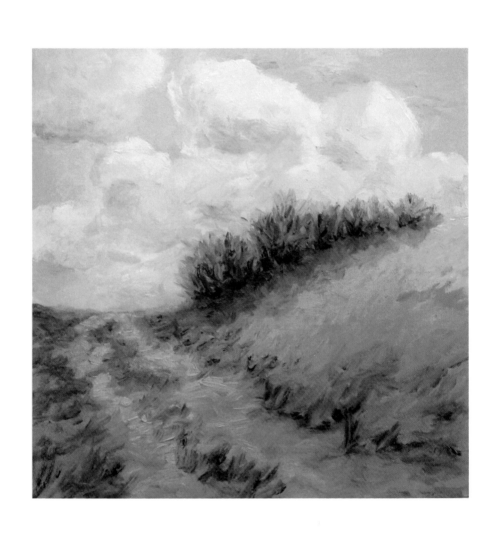

Three: Disposition

An account like the preceding one is compelling. It has an immediacy and relevance that draws us in. We gain better understanding of human emotions, fears and uncertainties. Our investment and participation are summoned. After reading or hearing this narrative, most of us would be happy to emulate the actions of the office nurse. She was of use. She knew what needed to be done. She acted kindly.

Generally, basic goals of kindness revolve around protecting and helping and being nice. Of course there are multiple manifestations of kindness. Sometimes kindness seems so basic as to appear ordinary—a gentle touch or caring expression. And sometimes a kindness can be utterly heroic, as when a person donates a kidney to a stranger.

In medicine, there are abundant opportunities for both small and great expressions of kindness. Certainly, kindness describes *how* clinicians should act. Most people accept that acting in a courteous and attentive manner toward another is part of being kind. But kindness is also intimately related to *what* clinicians do. And in illness care, this *what* usually focuses on efforts to protect and help—basic aims of kindness everywhere.

Today's healthcare is undergoing a revolution of sorts. There is heightened awareness of patient safety (protecting) and quality of care (helping). These goals constitute a roadmap directing *what* needs to be done for patients. Enhancing patient safety and quality of care can become definitive, tangible manifestations of kindness. Still, the *how* of our behavior very much reflects kindness as well. Patients don't always understand *what* we do for them, but they are acutely aware of *how* we treat them.

The narratives of this book attempt to demonstrate why the "how" and "what" of kindness should be an integral part of all illness care. They look at clinical work from the triad of safety, quality and acting kindly. These elements are inextricably intertwined and, in reality, all three comprise kindness in medicine. Stories reflect the nuances and impact of kindness in a more illuminating way than didactic analysis. Such narrative accounts can be easily recalled by a clinician and influence clinical behavior. A friend of mine described to me how his internist helps him manage his diabetes noting, "My doctor knows what to do and explains things." This physician's manner sounds simple and direct. She sounds kind.

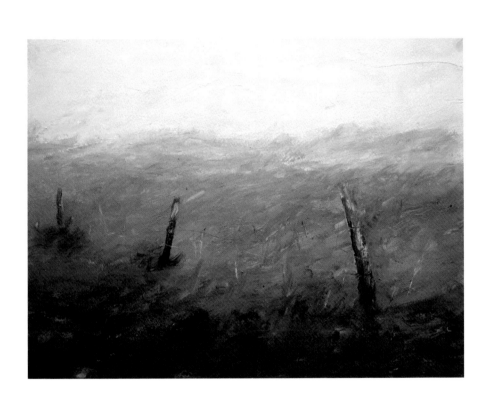

Four: Discovery

Most of us recall our best teachers. Many are memorable for being role models of kindness. The faculty for medical students and residents can have an enduring effect on future physicians. Some mentors may offer inspiring examples of clinical care. Unfortunately, others may come across as haughty and insensitive. I have vivid recollections of both types of interaction from my own training.

One incident I recall (and have repeated to my own students) involved a visiting professor from Cleveland. Frequently, such teaching sessions are an occasion for the visitor to display diagnostic acumen. But this esteemed clinician chose to focus on a common and frustrating occurrence—the patient who presents in crisis to an emergency department with physical complaints due to emotional turmoil. Such an event can be dramatic. For instance, the patient may have inability to speak or a paralysis that resembles a stroke. Almost always, the patient and family are unaware that this is due to an emotional crisis. Frequently, they are resistant to any explanation that implies the symptoms are not "real."

Physicians, for their part, can be dismissive of this type of patient, sometimes irritably suggesting that the individual is deliberately "faking" the problem. By implication, such patients lack a substantial illness like cancer or a heart attack. But this visiting professor urged students and residents to adopt a different perspective. He emphasized that any person who presents to an emergency department with such an emotional malady is indeed in crisis. He challenged us to take very seriously our obligation to listen intently, understand, respect and help such a patient. When I recount this professor's message for my current students, I am effectively sharing his narrative of kindness with another generation and beyond.

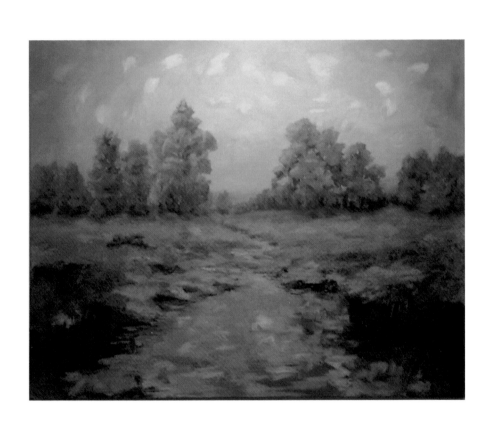

Five: Focus

Most commonly, kindness becomes real for people united in some form of relationship. Effective communication can play a crucial role, especially when medical issues are involved. I have a friend from Ireland whose speech seems quaint, at least by mid-America standards. When referring to her father with dementia, she noted that "he didn't particularly know anybody." On another occasion, my friend noted that her neighbor had "taken a stroke." To me, these phrases sound lyrical and her intent is evident.

But when I was a resident at a large inner city hospital in Kansas City, the meaning of certain phrases I encountered was not always so clear. Patients would often announce that they had the "miseries." That could include anemia, depression, a thyroid condition or a variety of other ailments. Another favored term was "falling out spells." This posed a thorny diagnostic challenge with possibilities including seizure, fainting or heart problems. Sorting these possibilities out meant carefully listening to the patient and prompting for further clarification.

Such focused effort is often required to achieve mutual understanding. This work of communication demonstrates why a clinician's goodwill alone is not sufficient. Successful engagement in another's story needs the commitment of active, resourceful listening followed by appropriate action.

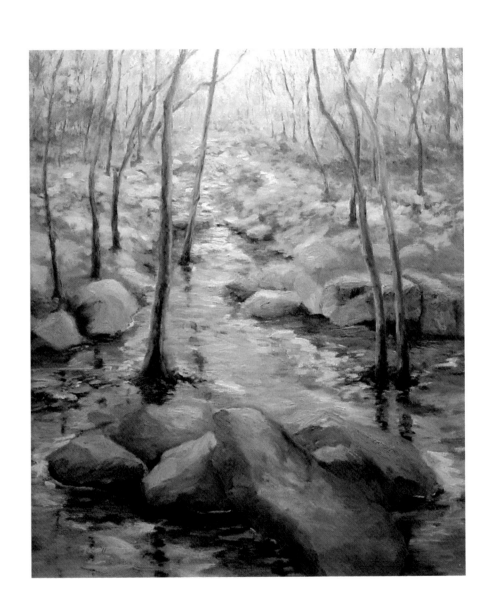

Six: Communication

Not surprisingly, the failure of a health professional to make certain a patient understands all communication can lead to safety issues. I recall one misunderstanding that seems almost humorous in retrospect but initially caused great consternation for the patient and family.

A sixty-one-year-old woman who'd had symptoms of Parkinson's disease for six years was on medication before each meal. Her tremor and rigidity were fairly well controlled during the day. However, her nights were miserable—she had leg stiffness and pain. It was difficult for her to arise to go the bathroom. I decided to add a long-acting medication at night to try to ease her symptoms and enable her to sleep better. She agreed with the proposal.

Three days later, she called the office sounding quite distraught. Her tremor had returned and she was so rigid that she could hardly walk. She insisted that she was taking her new nighttime medication properly. Her sudden worsening seemed most perplexing. Fortunately, my nurse methodically went through all of her medications with her, documenting how each was being taken. Only at that point did it become clear that the patient was confused about our instructions. Instead of simply adding the nocturnal Parkinson's medication and continuing her daytime doses, she substituted one for the other. She correctly took the nighttime dose, but stopped the daytime doses altogether. With this clarification, it was obvious why her Parkinson's symptoms so abruptly worsened during the day.

Both my nurse and I felt we had explained our initial treatment plan carefully. But such explanations are only sufficient if properly understood by the patient. Kindness is best served by tangible results, not just good intentions.

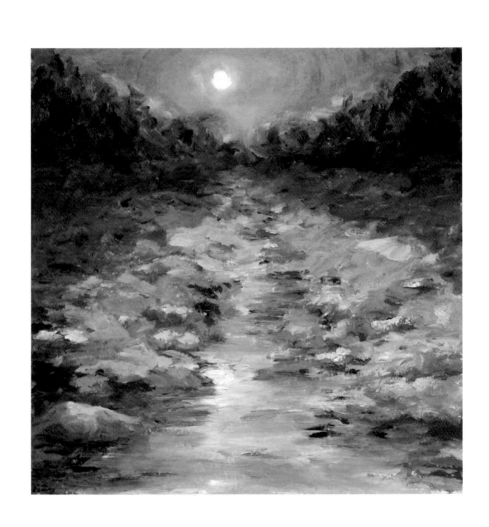

Seven: Resolve

The preceding story highlights how easy it is for patients to misunderstand instructions. But ineffective communication between clinicians can also put patients at risk, especially when it comes to medication errors. Current estimates suggest that one-third of patients entering a hospital are harmed in some fashion and medication errors are a major culprit.

A sixty-five-year-old man was hospitalized with a stroke. I recommended a blood thinner that has a risk of causing bleeding. This treatment must be monitored carefully with periodic blood tests and dosage adjustments. I ordered an initial dose for three days, assuming that subsequent dose changes would be made as needed. After the second hospital day, the patient was doing well and I indicated in the chart that I would not follow him daily. As it happened, on that same day, he was also transferred from the stroke unit to the rehabilitation unit at the direction of another physician. Upon transfer, my original three day drug order was recorded as being an ongoing daily dose. Also, inexplicably, the test to periodically check the effect of the drug was not ordered.

A week later, the patient's condition deteriorated and he was found to have bleeding in his brain. Lab testing confirmed that his blood was much thinner than required. As a result of this complication, his disability worsened.

When an error or bad event occurs in the hospital, there is an immediate tendency to point fingers indicating who is to blame. Often, unlikely coincidences seem to conspire to cause tragedy. The continuation of a blood thinner without lab monitoring would ordinarily have been recognized by nursing, pharmacy and clerical staff. And certainly the various physicians who periodically assessed him should have registered concern.

Experts in hospital safety emphasize that patient harm is usually not merely an error made by a single individual. Most adverse events are system failures in the institution's working environment. Often the culprit proves to be a breakdown in communication.

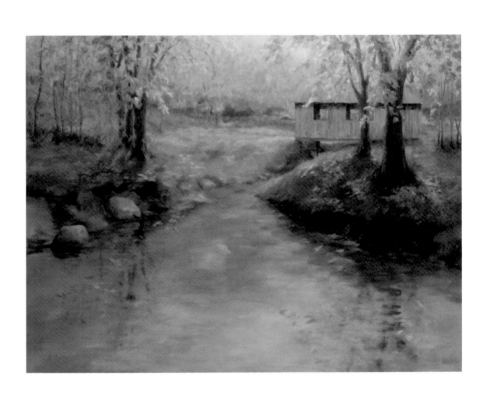

Eight: Distinction

The adverse events that cause injury to patients, while frequent, are merely the tip of an iceberg. Many mistakes and missteps end up being "close calls" but not actually harming someone. In the past, if an event did not cause harm, the clinicians involved would breathe a sigh of relief and move on. This might be characterized as an "ostrich approach" to safety. Fear of a malpractice action is often a factor in wanting to avoid analysis of close calls. But today's experts in health system safety stress the need for transparency and analysis of all such events.

Proving a negative, like reduction in risk, can be difficult. To the extent that a culture of safety exists in a hospital or clinic, real harm to patients is avoided. Although this work seems different from an overt act of kindness, the intent is the same.

Kindness has it deepest meaning and strongest force when it defines behaviors between individuals. Such activities might exist in the hospital, the workplace or in the home. While the impact of a kind act is readily evident, the language used to describe kindness may vary. A longtime family friend, Mead Bailey, was a keen observer of behavior and motivation. As his health problems mounted over several years, he had abundant opportunity to interact with nurses and doctors. Occasionally, he'd return from the hospital or clinic visit to announce that somebody he'd just met "had the magic." He might also use the term after being at the hardware store or buying groceries. For Mead, this compliment was unambiguous and understandable. He'd just encountered kindness.

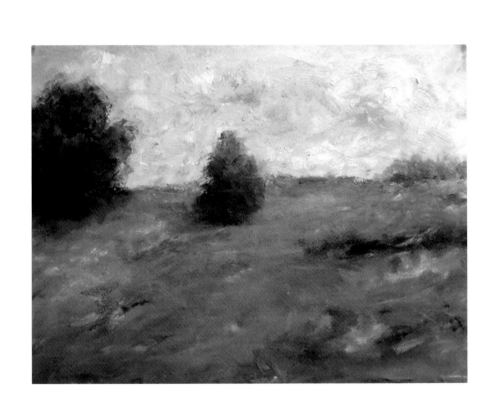

Nine: Advancement

Of course, all patients want medical treatment that works. When illness or injury strikes, a patient usually instinctively appeals for help. Most patients hope and presume that the doctors know what to do. Healthcare analysts use the term "quality of care" to characterize appropriate medical intervention. Frequently, quality is paired with safety as the essential goal for modern healthcare. Unfortunately, quality is not a universal reality—there are major regional variations in this country. Some parts of the United States do many more C-sections or carotid artery surgeries than others. Physicians may have uncertainty and disagreements about treatment options.

And to confound the issue even more, there are the patient's beliefs and wishes to consider. Clinicians may too readily focus on their own perceptions while failing to listen closely to the patient's viewpoint. This can be problematic because quality of care may well have more to do with a patient's perceived quality of life than with objective parameters for assessing a medical condition.

I am reminded of a sixty-five-year-old woman with Parkinson's disease. When she first came to see me, she was fearful that her new stiffness and tremor would force her to give up being principal organist for her church. She now takes pleasure in reminding me that, with treatment, she was able to continue playing the organ for another six years. For her, this was the most important measure of quality care. Issues like her gait stability and fall risk were secondary concerns.

Kindness comes into play most forcefully as a clinician focuses intently on the specifics of an individual's life. Kindness involves choices and endorses action. Often, the clinical interventions that result prove to be both pragmatic and hopeful.

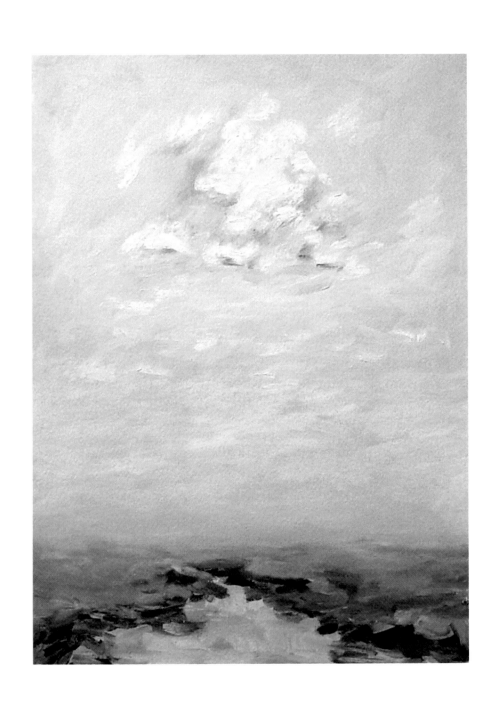

Ten: Healing

Quality healthcare is more than just an application of scientifically validated data. The manner in which the clinician interacts with the patient is also a pivotal factor in achieving high quality care. As an example, until recently there have been only four standard therapies for multiple sclerosis (MS). All involve injections with a frequency varying from daily to once a week. The drugs differ in subtle, but important, ways in terms of side effects and efficacy. I recall consulting on a twenty-five-year-old woman with a new diagnosis of MS. She wanted a second opinion. The first neurologist she had seen did a thorough evaluation and established the correct diagnosis. After reviewing the tests with her, this physician gave her literature on the four MS therapies, suggesting that she read about each and decide which one she wanted to take.

This woman found the first physician's approach unsettling. She intuitively knew that she needed more direction. The first clinician failed to provide advice she needed and expected. Even if the patient devoted considerable time toward researching the four therapies for MS, she could still lack the experience and acumen to choose which one is best for her. The drugs are not identical and her personal circumstances might well magnify the significance of certain side effects. As she confronts the reality of this chronic illness, she may be apprehensive and distracted. She could well have difficulty making a comparative analysis of possible treatments.

A physician should carefully provide her with relevant options. But in the end, I believe, the doctor owes it to the patient to offer a recommendation as to which therapy seems most suitable. It can be perceived by the patient as basically unkind to not offer such guidance and support.

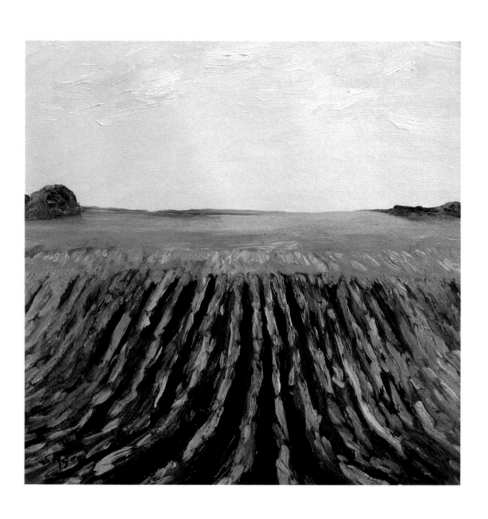

Eleven: Rescue

The safety and quality movement promises to transform the model for delivery of healthcare in this country. Patient welfare is the focus of these innovations. As noted earlier, safety and quality may be thought of as the *what* of medicine. But, as demonstrated by the woman debating MS therapies, *how* clinicians provide care is equally important. Again, the interconnection between safety, quality and kindness is evident.

Several years ago, I encountered a very effective way to think about the *what* and *how* of clinical care. A healthcare consulting firm had posted on its website the photograph of a young girl accompanied by the poignant appeal "Don't hurt me. Heal me. Be nice to me." Any patient faced with serious illness or injury could voice a similar hope. I find this entreaty stunning in its simplicity and universality. The entreaty "Don't hurt me" pleads for safety. "Heal me" pertains to quality of care. And "Be nice to me" is a simple request for kind interaction.

Recently, I was discussing the foregoing triad with two fourth year medical students. One of the students recalled the time when his mother became suddenly ill and was found to have widespread cancer. He was a junior in college and planning on medical school. As the only living relative, he met with his mother's oncologist. The student perceived this physician to be detached and unfeeling. He was told during their brief visit that the cancer was too advanced for treatment and that "nothing could be done." The medical student emphasized that this exchange with the physician was very disappointing and unsettling. As a result, he began to question his own career choice and decided not to enter medical school after college. Two years later, after much soul searching, he returned to his original plan. He stressed that that hurtful encounter dramatically altered the type of physician he'll strive to be.

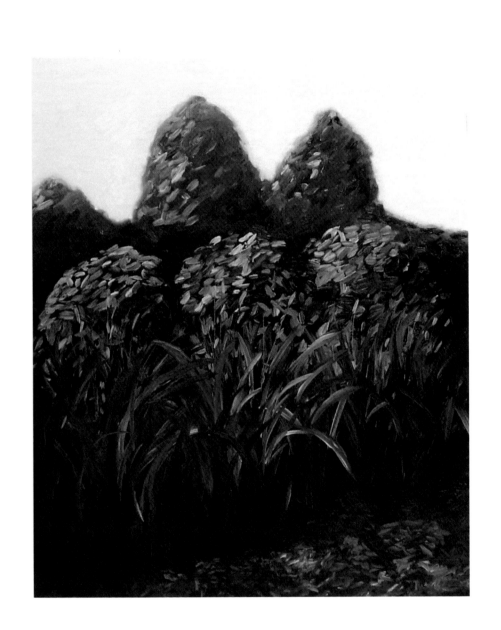

Twelve: Passion

In the hospital, we generally think of decisive action coming from the principles, the doctors or nurses. On the other hand, for the medical student, or any student, there is often a sense of merely "treading water." It seems as if real life will begin after graduation or at some other dimly perceived future date. Somehow student life does not feel like the real thing.

To counter this perception, I have frequently told my students about Ms Murphy. As a fourth year medical student, Ms Murphy opted to spend several weeks on my clinical service. One of our patients was a seventy-two-year-old man with severe weakness from a spinal cord inflammation. We managed his care during his acute hospital stay and then followed his slow progress on the rehabilitation unit. While I assessed him only periodically during the latter stages of his hospital stay, I was aware that Ms Murphy visited him daily.

When this patient was ready for discharge from the hospital, Ms Murphy and I stopped by his hospital room to say good-bye. The patient expressed gratitude to me for my clinical expertise. I too thought I had done a very good job. He then surprised us both by turning to the medical student and emotionally thanking her, declaring, "But Ms Murphy you saved my life."

To this day, I am moved by what this student accomplished, just beyond my view. On the one hand, she was merely a student. She made no major diagnostic decisions or treatment adjustments. But Ms Murphy was unwaveringly present for this patient on a daily basis. She listened to his fears and frustrations. Above all, she was kind.

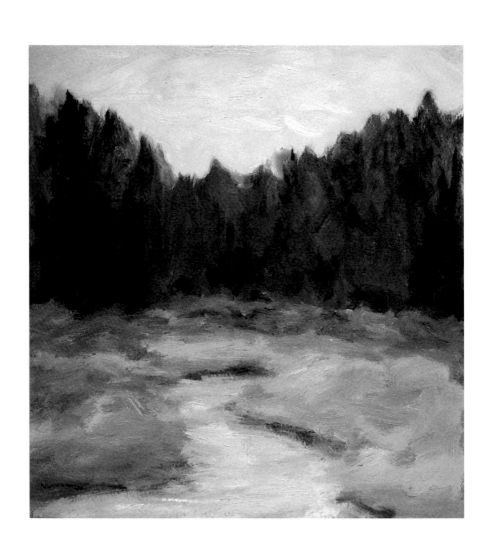

Thirteen: Family

Picture a fatigued physician holding a vigil with distraught parents at the bedside of a sick child. Or imagine a gentle nurse carefully repositioning a gravely ill, elderly person in a hospital bed. Such images reside in our collective understanding of how illness care should be provided. In real life, kindness can be more complex than our cherished stereotypes of optimal illness care. There may be differences of opinion and sometimes adversarial confrontations. Fortunately, many disagreements can be resolved over time by consensus.

Some years ago, I cared for an active seventy-five-year-old male who was discovered in an unresponsive state. Over the next two days, extensive testing failed to reveal the cause for his coma. On the morning of the third hospital day, I was approached by his wife and four children who seemed united in their opinion that all treatment should be stopped. They felt certain that the patient would not want to survive in a compromised state and would not want aggressive care.

I was uneasy about stopping supportive treatment. Testing had not shown a major stroke or any other irreversible condition. The assembled family and I had a lengthy discussion but remained divided as to what to do. Finally, I bartered for a compromise. We agreed to treat aggressively for two more days and then stop treatment if there was no improvement. After that interval, the patient seemed slightly improved and the family consented to an extension of treatment for another two days. We then agreed on further increments of time-limited care. After about a week, the patient began to improve rapidly and awoke in Rip Van Winkle fashion.

Of course, everyone was thrilled with this patient's unexpected recovery. He was able to continue an energetic involvement in his community for another five years. But I remain humbled by the fact that none of the physicians who cared for him knew what caused his coma. At times, it seems, humility can be an ally of kindness.

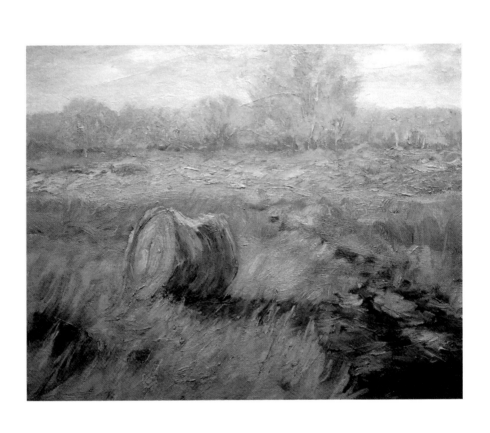

Fourteen: Probability

Unfortunately, in today's illness care, patients and families often sense a lack of basic kindness and concern. Sometimes uncertainty about prognosis may shade their view. But other issues can also intrude. Conversations overheard in hospital cafeterias or hallways may reveal disillusionment and anger. Seemingly interminable waiting for needed testing and subsequent results is common. Comments are made about how much time nurses and doctors spend working with computers rather than at the bedside providing patient care. Often, I think, patients and families perceive the healthcare team as being too busy and preoccupied. Such dissatisfactions, at their core, seem to boil down to a perceived lack of kindness.

In truth, most patients and families seem just as concerned about *how* care is given as they are with *what* is done and accomplished. Indeed, when a patient and family are treated in a kind manner, they often seem inordinately grateful. Their appreciation frequently far exceeds the effort expended by the clinician. In times of illness and fragility, the impact of kindness seems magnified. Basic kindness in healthcare does not really differ from kindness extended in any of life's social situations. But in the face of serious illness, the ground seems to shift and perspective is altered. The need for kindness is most urgent.

Of course, there are instances when a clinician simply can't deliver what a patient believes is warranted. I am reminded of a fifty-two-year-old plumber who came to me with a headache of two months duration. He recalled hitting his head forcefully on a pipe several months earlier. Testing revealed a brain tumor. He and his wife were convinced that treatment for the tumor should be covered under his workman's compensation policy. To their way of thinking, he was perfectly fine until he hit his head on the pipe and developed headaches. Surely, they argued, his brain tumor was due to this on-the-job trauma. Despite my repeated explanations that head trauma does not produce a tumor, this couple remained undeterred in their contention that he deserved a workman's compensation claim.

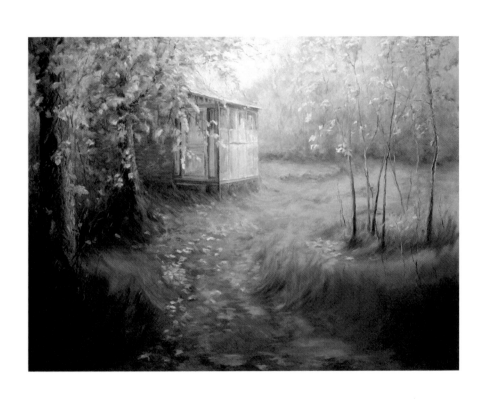

Fifteen: Yearning

Sometimes patients don't view efforts to ensure safety and quality as being kind. Opinions may vary as to appropriate treatment options. Often anecdotal claims for remedies circulate among patients and families seeking a cure for a chronic illness. I have especially found this to be the case with multiple sclerosis (MS). Over the years, the internet and other sources have touted various remedies which have no demonstrable scientific benefit. These treatments have included bee pollen, bee stings, bovine colostrums, removal of fillings in teeth, hyperbaric oxygen therapy and various other nonprescription integrative therapies. Patients have fiercely defended and endorsed all of these remedies despite the warranted skepticism and concern of clinicians and scientists.

Recently, there has been much interest in a so-called "liberation therapy" devised by an Italian neurologist. He reported that chronic cerebrospinal venous insufficiency (CCSVI) was the cause of MS. Supposedly, narrowing of the veins leading from the brain was the culprit. Techniques to dilate jugular veins by stents and angioplasty were recommended. A number of my patients have been interested in this CCSVI therapy.

A thirty-year-old woman was especially insistent. Her MS was fairly mild and she was doing well on standard MS therapy. But she wanted me to endorse CCSVI treatment for her. She had done an enormous amount of reading on this subject and was in internet communication with others who felt just as strongly that this treatment was valuable. No amount of discussion and reasoning with her altered her opinion. When I pointed out that the treatment was speculative, had not been proven and has some potentially serious risks, she seemed to argue for it all the more fiercely. She *knew* this therapy would work and she wanted the healthcare system to provide it for her. She even consulted with a local vascular surgeon who told her a vein procedure could be performed if I would only sanction it.

Ultimately, this patient left my practice. Over the two years since I last saw her, there have been a number of scientific studies that have conclusively shown that CCSVI does not work. Researchers have urged that the therapy not be used. But I still feel badly about how angry this patient became with me when I would not endorse this treatment. From a safety and quality of care standpoint, I certainly feel I did the right thing. But I'm quite sure this patient believes I was not kind to her because I didn't provide what she was requesting. My being right doesn't erase the memory of her recriminations. The author Oscar Wilde observed, "The truth is rarely pure and never simple." The same can sometimes be said for kindness.

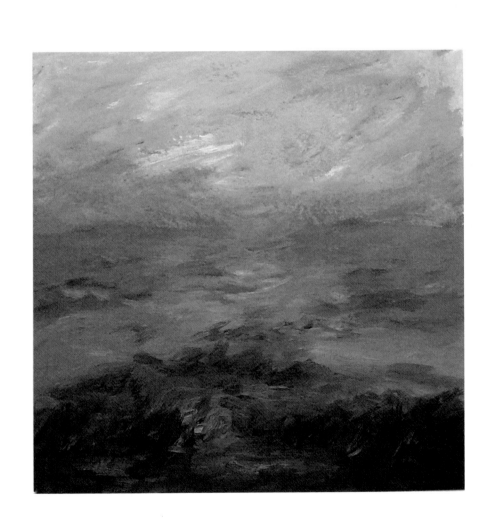

Sixteen: Courage

On occasion, kindness requires departing from the normal script. I had evaluated a forty-five-year-old male with new headaches. Because I was concerned about his history, I scheduled an MRI for the next day. As I was giving an out-of-town lecture the following morning, I asked him to come to the office in the late afternoon to meet with me. This fellow was understandably apprehensive about his test result and came to my office just before noon. My nurse again explained that I was teaching and would return to visit with him later in the day. At that point he said to my nurse, "I know you have the scan results and I want to be told now. I think I have cancer." As the patient correctly surmised, the nurse did in fact have the MRI report from the radiologist. And it did confirm the presence of a tumor.

This nurse, who had worked in neurology for many years, faced a thorny dilemma. Nursing ordinarily never reveals a serious diagnosis—it is left to the physician to handle. But she felt she couldn't lie to the patient and imply that the test had not yet been interpreted. The nurse also felt it would be cruel to force this patient to wait several more hours for confirmation of what he already feared and suspected.

After considering these options, the nurse sat down with him and gently explained that the MRI did show a tumor. She talked generally about the next diagnostic steps that would take place and tried to comfort him. By the time I arrived to visit with him, he understood the seriousness of his situation. He'd had time to formulate other questions he wished to address with me. And he expressed gratitude to the nurse for understanding his situation and caring about him.

In the world of medicine, we often invoke the term "professionalism" to describe clinical behavior. Professionalism specifically places emphasis on what motivates a physician or nurse to act appropriately. In addition to invoking values like compassion and empathy, terms like integrity and respect are emphasized. But all these attributes of professionalism are subjective and potentially variable. What determines if the nurse has sufficient compassion for the man with the brain tumor? She may feel sorry for him, but still refuse to provide information until the physician arrives.

From my perspective, her actions were compassionate and appropriate in this exceptional situation. She had done what kindness required. Kindness here is not what the nurse *feels* but what she *does*.

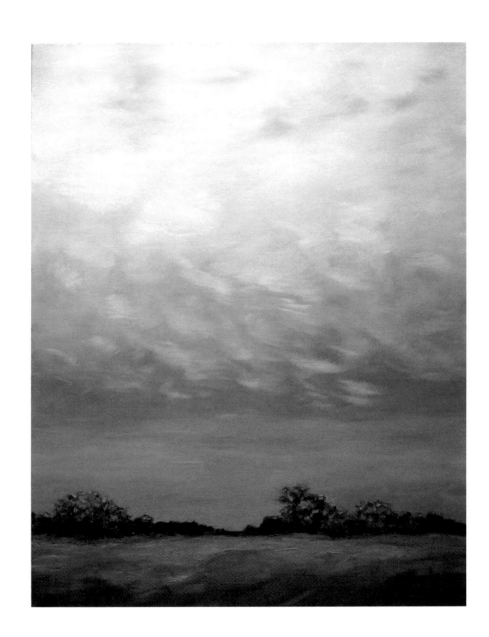

Seventeen: Cooperation

While the major emphasis in healthcare appropriately centers upon the clinician/patient interaction, it warrants noting that clinicians often fail to treat each other with respect and kindness. The nurse, in the preceding story, could have been reprimanded by clinic administration for operating "out of scope" for nursing practice. Some physicians may have berated her for usurping a doctor's authority to reveal a diagnosis. Such responses would presume that maintaining normal office protocol should trump making an exception for an individual patient. Sadly, it is not uncommon for a physician or nurse to complain that colleagues fail to show basic consideration. This problem seems to be escalating. In many healthcare institutions there are heavy workloads and frustrating time constraints. Fatigue often contributes to poor behavior as well.

The times I recall acting unkindly with colleagues are like thorns of memory that continue to prick long after the incident. I remember a 2:00 AM call from a charge nurse informing me that one of my patients, a seventy-five-year-old woman with a stroke, had fallen off the toilet and injured her hip. I was immediately angry, partly at being awakened for the third time that night, and blurted out, "how could you have let this happen?" When I arrived at the hospital, I was still upset and in the mood for recriminations, especially when I learned that the patient had fractured her hip and needed surgery. My behavior was embarrassing. When I calmed down, I learned that the nursing staff had been trying hard all night to protect the patient. Although her weakness from the stroke was fairly mild, two staff had assisted her to the bathroom. Once situated, she had then been very insistent that she be left alone "for some privacy." The patient acknowledged that she fell off the toilet when she impulsively reached for an object on the floor.

Realistically, those nurses could not have foreseen or prevented the accident. For me to assign blame by my words and demeanor was unkind and unwarranted. Any time clinicians experience a lack of kindness and respect from colleagues, teamwork suffers. Nursing and I shared the same goals for this patient. Too late, I remembered we were teammates, not adversaries.

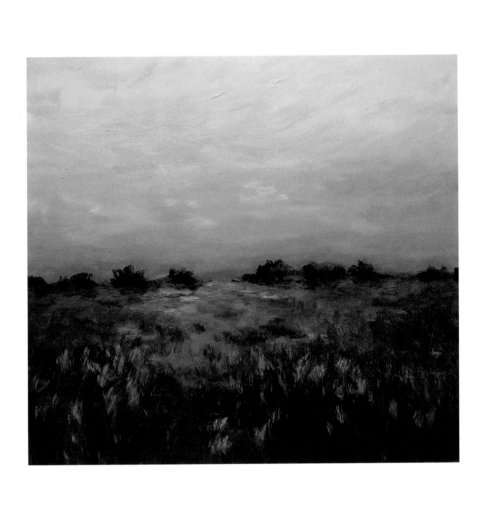

Eighteen: Consequence

Medicine is stressful and demanding. Clinicians can be worn down by the demands of long hours, the complexity of decision making and fear of mistakes. Such factors can contribute to tensions between clinical colleagues and seemingly uncaring, capricious behavior toward patients.

Sometimes a patient's unadorned account of the dysfunction in the healthcare system is just what is needed to shake up the status quo. A specific example can remind us that rationalization for inappropriate behavior does not constitute sufficient justification for it.

One Thursday, I was having coffee with a friend who confided that she'd just had an abdominal CAT scan that morning to evaluate unexplained weight loss. She was fearful that something bad would be discovered and she'd called her physician's office shortly after the test to inquire when she would receive the results. She was informed that her physician was out of town for the rest of the week and would provide her with the CAT scan test result on Monday. My friend balked at the delay and requested that one of her physician's colleagues provide the result. She was informed that it was against office policy for physicians in the group to provide potentially sensitive test results to another partner's patient.

A four-day wait to receive the result of a major test seems unconscionable. I suspect most clinicians and lay people would agree on this score. And yet, over the years, I've occasionally heard similar ineffectual explanations given to patients in an effort to justify "the way things are done."

In medicine, as well as many other social and commercial endeavors, the implications of policies and procedures may not always be fully apparent. Probably each of us has experienced frustration at seemingly inflexible rules. But medicine needs to be held to a uniquely high standard. Patients are not detached consumers of an optional commodity. In those times of potentially serious illness, patients are vulnerable and dependent. Often they feel overwhelmed and powerless. They need and deserve the kindness of those who control the levers of illness care.

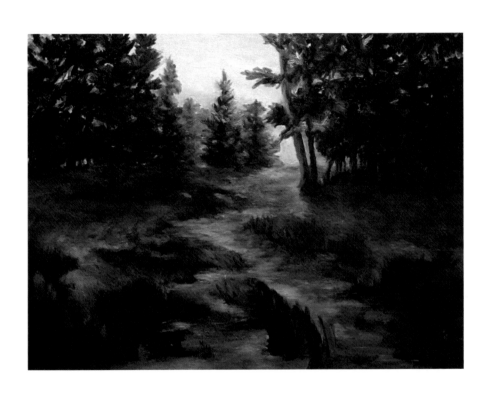

Nineteen: Covenant

Narrative accounts, such as those used in this volume, can enrich our understanding of illness care and kindness. Indeed, throughout recorded history, story has been used as a means to understand the forces impacting upon human lives. Noble stories can inspire, but tales of shortcomings can be effectively illustrative as well. Often patients and families find the healthcare system to be daunting. Many who pass through the portal of illness care are dissatisfied, at least in part.

There is a paradox here. The physician and nurse, as well as others in healthcare, have special training and abilities to heal. And yet, somehow, the good intentions of clinicians are often squandered in the mechanics of healthcare delivery. Many are disillusioned. I know nurses who have opted to leave clinical work after several years for employment elsewhere. And medical students have recounted conversations with practicing physicians who declare that if they were just beginning a career, they would not choose to go into medicine.

Perhaps clinicians need to be challenged to view their profession as a solemn calling. And clinicians, as well as patients, should be reminded that seeking illness care is fundamentally different from engaging in other commercial transactions. It has to be. The clinician cannot be a mere salesperson. The clinician has special knowledge and influence, while the patient is inherently vulnerable because of illness and thus dependent on the clinician's good will. If a physician recommends costly treatment or painful therapy, most patients assume it is for their own good.

This dynamic relationship demands a solemn agreement, a covenant as it were, between clinician and patient. By virtue of being a healthcare professional, the clinician must feel duty-bound to provide each patient with safety, quality and kindness. And, under the auspices of this triad, every patient deserves to hope and expect that appropriate care will be provided.

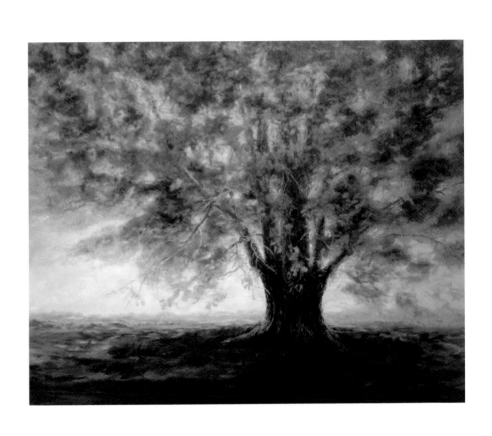

Twenty: Panorama

Definitions of kindness can take you so far, but not all the way. A descriptive analysis can fail to capture the spontaneity and gentleness that may underlie a kind act. Also, aspects like intention and self-sacrifice are hard to fold into a succinct definition of kindness. It is, I believe, virtually impossible to define the myriad of ways kindness can illumine human interactions. Kindness is familiar. We all recognize it. Kindness is a disposition that needs to be cultivated. It is not an attribute that is somehow bestowed or guaranteed.

The far-reaching impact of an intended kindness may be completely unforeseen at the time it is offered. And despite good intentions, each of us is at risk of acting unkindly. Those times when we do act unkindly are disheartening. But such instances can also serve as sentinel reminders of who we really want to be.

This book is not intended to be a comprehensive analysis of kindness. In some ways, kindness may be so fundamental as to defy scholarly analysis. It seems akin to trying to critique the Golden Rule. Stories of personal relationships work better. My emphasis on safety and quality has, by intention, been narrowly focused. And I have deliberately worked to demonstrate that kindness involves specifics—the *what*, as well as the *how*, of medicine.

In virtually every walk of life, individuals can figure out ways to be kind. Kindness is universal and necessary. The impact of kind actions endures in people's memories and narratives. The kindness extended by clinicians in healthcare is similar to kind behavior anywhere. Stories in this collection can serve as prototypical examples of what kindness might mean in all aspects of people's lives. Location and occupation are not critical variables—opportunities abound in small communities as well as in large metropolitan centers.

Acts of kindness must be intended and implemented on a case by case basis, one person at a time, over and over again. Pondering kind thoughts is not sufficient. Our challenge is choosing to *act* kindly. At the most basic level, kind actions revolve around protecting, helping and being nice. Opportunities for kindness may be fleeting. At times, we may have only a limited window of possibility. Vigilance and focus are required, but acting kindly is not an elusive objective. It is concrete, attainable and worth the effort, for each of us.

References and Sources

Bellow, Saul. *The Adventures of Augie March*. The Viking Press, 1953

Freeman, J.W. *The Colors of Care*. Ex Machina Publishing Company, 2005 (Chap 10 "Being There" adapted and used in Chap 2)

Freeman, J. W. "Kindness and the Clinician" from DeGroot Center for Ethics and Caring Newsletter, Fall 2011

Freeman, J.W. "Is Premier Health Care Our Goal?", South Dakota Medicine, Feb 2011

Freeman, J.W. and Hoffman, W.W. "Kindness in Medicine: Appeal and Promise", South Dakota Medicine, Sept 2011

Healthcare Performance Improvement (HPI) (internet).(PowerPoint file), Building a Culture of Safety. Available from:http://hpiresults.com. (Source of "Don't hurt me, heal me, be nice to me").Accessed May 2008 and used in essay ("Is Premier Health Care Our Goal?") in South Dakota Medicine, Feb 2011

Wilde, Oscar. *The Importance of Being Earnest*. Bernhard Tauchnitz, 1910

Paintings in Order of Presentation

Cover: Great Egret Along
    the James River
Forward: Prairie Sentry
1 Dakota Sky
2 Rain Soaked
3 Country Road
4 Windy Day
5 Prairie Passage
6 Freeman's Creek
7 Meandering, Series
8 Covered Bridge
9 Prairie Rough
10 Prairie Sky, Series
11 Pasture's Edge, Series
12 Garden Path
13 Gray Sky along the
    Mickelson Trail, II
14 Pasture's Edge, Series
15 Cabin in the Hollow
16 Sun Series, I
17 Prairie Sky, Series
18 Pasture's Edge, Series
19 Along the Mickelson Trail, Series
20 Prairie Sentry, II

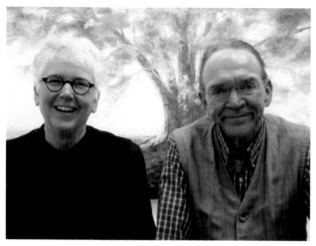
Sheila Agee and Jerome Freeman

About the Author

Jerome W. Freeman, MD is a practicing neurologist and educator. He is professor and chair of the Department of Neurosciences at Sanford School of Medicine. He has taught bioethics to medical students and undergraduates for many years. Dr. Freeman has a special interest in the use of literature to understand illness and treatment issues. He is the founding director of the DeGroot Center at Sanford USD Medical Center in Sioux Falls, SD. The Center, which is dedicated to education in bioethics, humanities and the healing arts, is currently celebrating its 25th anniversary year. His previous publications include three volumes of poetry and two collections of essays dealing with issues of illness care—*The Colors of Care: What are Those Doctors Thinking?* (2005) and *Come and See* (1995). He also co-authored an anthology focused on issues of caring, *The Call to Care*, in 1999. Dr. Freeman and his wife, Mary, live on the rolling prairie of eastern South Dakota.

About the Artist

Sheila Agee works out of her studio in the country near Brandon, South Dakota. Some of the works in this book were painted from images found on Dr. Freeman's land, such as the "Cabin in the Hollow" and the "Covered Bridge." Sheila works 'plein air' and from photographs, but finds it best to quickly abandon the restraints of the original image and just paint.

CPSIA information can be obtained
at www.ICGtesting.com
Printed in the USA
LVIC01n1959101213
364139LV00003BC/21